Affirmations FOR Family CAREGIVERS

HARRIET HODGSON

Georgia

Published by WriteLife Publishing

(an imprint of Boutique of Quality Books Publishing Company)

www.writelife.com

Printed in the United States of America

Cover photo from www.istockphoto.com.
Author Photo by Haley Earley
Cover design by Ellis Dixon

ISBN 978-1-60808-146-2 (p)
ISBN 978-1-60808-147-9 (e)

Library of Congress Control Number: 2015939447

For more information about this busy author and grandmother, visit www.harriethodgson.com.
To contact the author personally, send an email to harriethodgson@charter.net.

Books in the Family Caregiver Series

The Family Caregiver's Guide
Published by WriteLife Publishing in September 2015

Affirmations for Family Caregivers
Published by WriteLife Publishing in September 2015

A Journal for Family Caregivers
Publishing Date - March 2016

Contents

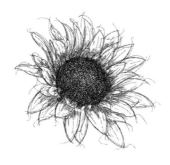

Features of This Book

Caregivers don't have much time for reading. You may feel lucky if you have time to read a magazine article, let alone a book. I know how pressed for time you can be, and that's why this book is designed for easy reading. Features include:

- **Organized by topic.** Each of these topics explores many subtopics, issues you deal with on a daily basis, such as self-care, responsibility, quiet time, routine, etc. When you need a boost, you need it now. Turn to the chapter that matches your need and read some of the affirmations.

- **Friendly layout.** Crowding affirmations together demeans the affirmations and causes eyestrain. You'll notice that each page has white space that respects the affirmations and provides places for your eyes to rest. You may also use the white space to jot down notes about the affirmations.

- **Experienced-based.** I've been a family caregiver for eighteen years, and there are many years to come. Though the affirmations come from my experience, I think you will find they apply to your experience. You may find yourself muttering, "That happened to me" or "I agree with that."

- **Informative.** Many affirmations contain information, such as a definition, or symptoms, or resources for caregivers. Though you may have already considered these things, the affirmations serve as reminders.

- **Adaptable.** These affirmations are written for family caregivers, yet they may apply to paid caregivers as well. Family and paid caregivers share many common tasks. Over time, paid caregivers may think of their long-term clients as family, and clients may return this feeling.

- **Present-day approach.** Most affirmation writing experts tell you to use the present tense to write about the life you hope to have. Affirmations about the future you hope to have, although you write them in the present tense, are really goals. One problem with that approach is that you may miss the positives of your current life. The affirmations in this book come from the author's life.

- **Affirmation writing tips.** If you've never done any writing, the idea of writing affirmations may seem intimidating. Don't worry. The writing tips in this book will get you started. There are also practice pages for you to write affirmations that support your caregiving.

Introduction

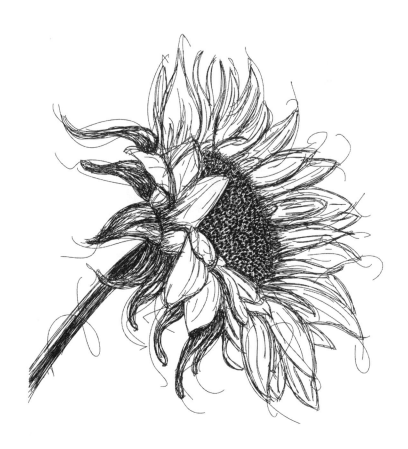

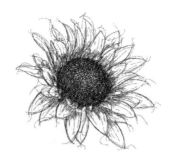

I never dreamed I would be my mother's family caregiver, but that's what happened.

The funny, kind, witty mother of my childhood started to have mini-strokes. She had her first mini-stroke the day of my father's funeral. My aunt, who had been staying with my mother, attributed my mother's confusion to "sleeping hard." As the months passed, my mother's intelligence started to slip, probably the result of more strokes. Her judgment slipped, too. Without telling anyone, she contacted a mover, left her house, and boarded a plane to Florida so she could be near her older sister. Family members were shocked to learn she was gone.

Moving proved to be one of the worst decisions of my mother's life. I called her regularly and became aware of her dwindling intelligence. One day my mother called me to tell me she had been found wandering around a department store, looking for her car. The sales associate told my mother, "Cars are parked outside the store, not inside." Mom told the story in a controlled manner and reacted calmly when I told her she needed to move to Rochester, Minnesota, to be close to family support.

I contacted a mover and found an apartment for her, and my husband and I set a date to drive to Florida and pick up my mother. Unfortunately, she called again to tell me she wasn't going to move. First, I tried reasoning with my mother, and that didn't work. Finally, I resorted to blunt truth. "You called to tell me you were found wandering in a department store. This isn't safe, and you aren't safe." There was silence on the other end of the phone.

Then I heard a deep sigh of resignation, and my mother said, "All right. I'll come."

Looking back now, I realize my job as a family caregiver "officially" began that day. I moved my mother from her large apartment into a studio apartment to conserve funds. Every day I did something for my mother. I made medical and dental appointments for her, took her out to lunch every Wednesday, ran errands on weekdays, cooked a gourmet dinner for her every Sunday, managed her finances, and represented her in a class-action lawsuit when I discovered she had been defrauded of $50,000.

This went on for nine years, and I didn't realize how exhausted I was until my mother died. I resumed my community activities and became involved in new ones. Life was good, and I was coasting along. But on a snowy February night in 2007, my elder daughter died from the injuries she received in a car crash. Two days later, on the same weekend, my father-in-law succumbed to pneumonia. Eight weeks later, my brother and only sibling died of a heart attack. In the fall of the same year, my twin grandchildren's father died from the injuries he received in another car crash. His death made my twin grandchildren orphans, and my husband and I became their guardians.

I never dreamed I would be my grandchildren's guardian and caregiver.

The twins were fifteen years old when they moved in with us. Suddenly, our quiet lives were transformed by the busyness of teenage years. We attended gymnastics meets, choir concerts, marching band concerts, high school plays, and school meetings. I cooked meals the twins would like, shared recipes, stocked up on snacks for sleepovers, and tried to catch up on teen lingo. I learned a few words, but they weren't enough to keep up with daily events.

Somehow, and I wasn't sure how, I had to figure out how to grieve for four family members and stay upbeat for the twins. I grieved for those I'd lost, and I grieved for the twins and the terrible tragedies they had suffered. As weeks became months and months became years, we slowly melded into a family. Being the twins' caregiver turned into one of the most meaningful experiences of my life. Caregiving was my new mission, and it was a sacred one. Both twins graduated from high school with honors. Though they left for college, I stayed involved in their lives.

I sent them goodie packages, cooked their favorite meals when they came home, and shared my expertise when asked. The twins also shared their expertise with me. My granddaughter is a talented photographer and a gifted writer. I asked for her opinion on many potential cover photographs. My grandson is a technical whiz and helps me whenever I need it. I would be lost without his help. While the twins were in college, I think their appreciation of home grew. Though I can't prove this, both of them were excited to come home during college breaks.

Life settled down a bit and returned to normal. Then, in October of 2013, my husband's aorta dissected. I drove him to the hospital, and the emergency team gave him medication for pain, but it didn't stop the bleeding, and my husband was quickly bleeding to death. Surgeons operated on him twice in a desperate attempt to save his life. Still, his internal bleeding continued, and doctors were pumping blood into him as fast as he was losing it. Finally, the lead physician gave my husband a choice: bleed to death or undergo drastic surgery. My husband chose the surgery option because he wanted to see his grandkids graduate from college.

Though the surgeons saved my husband's life, he suffered a spinal stroke during the surgery, and his legs are now paralyzed.

I never dreamed I would be my husband's caregiver.

He was institutionalized for eight months: one in the Intensive Care Unit, then back to the ICU because of wound problems, later transferred to rehabilitation, and finally sent to a nursing home for wound care and physical therapy. On June 30, 2014, my husband was released to my care. Because I have cared for three generations of family members, I understand what is involved, the challenges caregivers face, the up days and down days. I know how fatigue can alter thinking, that lack of sleep affects behavior. To share some of the things I learned and broaden my understanding, I wrote *The Family Caregiver's Guide*. I also became a contributing writer for The Caregiver Space website.

Usually I am an even-keeled person with a ready sense of humor, a willingness to learn; and I'm just plain persistent. Some days, however, caring for my disabled husband strained my patience and resolve. "I need a boost," I said to myself. "What will it be?" Several weeks later, the answer to this question came to me—write affirmations for caregivers. This was an easy answer because I had written a collection of affirmations for bereaved people. Writing affirmations for caregivers was a logical follow-up, something I could do for myself and for others. After you have read some of my affirmations, I hope you will start writing your own.

There are many benefits of affirmation writing. First, it helps you switch negative thoughts to positive ones. Second, you become more aware of the blessings in your life. Third, affirmations can act as mini pep talks and give you energy boosts when you need them. You may wish to highlight your favorite affirmations. I have a particular favorite: Caregiving is a journey, and love is my guide. I think of this affirmation every day. Post some affirmations that "speak" to you on the refrigerator door. Write an affirmation on a small piece of paper and stick it in your pocket. Share some of your favorite affirmations with friends.

The affirmations in this book may cause you to evaluate your caregiving, search for information, sign up for a course, participate in online education, join a support group, participate in an online community, take surprising steps, and even rethink your life. Whether you're a reluctant caregiver, an eager caregiver, or an appointed one, you're a caregiver now, and it's one of the hardest, most rewarding jobs in the world. Life is changing right before your eyes, and you're adapting constantly. Hard as this may be, keep in mind that you are making a difference in someone's life. Kudos to you!

CHAPTER 1

My Caregiving Tasks

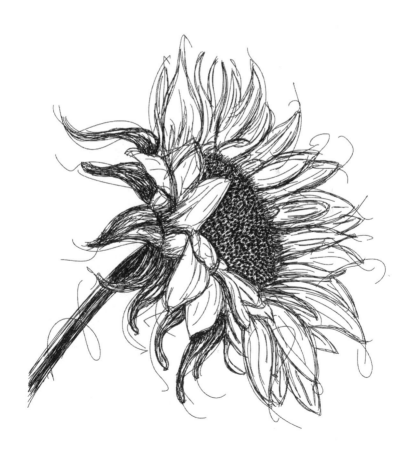

Each morning I awaken with a sense of purpose.

—⚮—

Attentive listening is a gift for my loved one and a gift for me.

—⚮—

Bad days (and all caregivers have them) often occur
because of lack of sleep.

—⚮—

Every day is a jewel in the necklace of life, and I will remember
these days when my task is done.

—⚮—

Planning is key to good caregiving, and I involve my loved one
in planning as much as possible.

—⚮—

I grant my loved one's wishes—a favorite meal, good books to read,
watching television together—and this is a joy.

Assessing my loved one's needs is an ongoing task.

—⁂—

I'm not afraid to try new things, make mistakes, admit them,
and learn from them.

—⁂—

I'm my loved one's advocate and accept the responsibilities
that come with this task.

—⁂—

Changes in plans don't throw me off balance; they activate
my coping skills.

—⁂—

Being a family caregiver doesn't erase the need for courtesy and tact.

—⁂—

Caregiving experience teaches me as much, maybe more,
than any course I take.

Past caregiving experience applies to current experience
in surprising ways.

—⚡—

Every job has its messy aspects, and that makes me appreciate
the non-messy aspects more.

—⚡—

Caregiving generates lots of paperwork, and I file information
as soon as it arrives.

—⚡—

I give myself permission to be a non-perfectionist.

—⚡—

When I'm at the grocery store, I stock up on caregiving supplies
to save another trip.

—⚡—

I had to give up on some things to become a caregiver, and that's okay.

I continue to learn about caregiving, a process that helps
my loved one and me.

—⚍—

Today is a good day to try something new.

—⚍—

There is a wealth of caregiving information on the Internet, but I'm
selective about the websites I visit and what I read.

—⚍—

Becoming a caregiver links me with 65+ million other
family caregivers in America. Wow!

—⚍—

Becoming a caregiver has altered my self-concept, and it is
greater than before.

—⚍—

Because surprise visitors can throw off our daily routine,
I prepare for them.

Though I don't know what the future holds, I can prepare for it
by sorting possessions, updating legal documents,
and making sure bills are paid.

—∞—

Helping my loved one set new goals is one of my tasks.

—∞—

Caregiving is a balancing act between my loved one's dependence and
need for independence.

—∞—

Whenever possible, I give my loved one choices so he or she
can retain a sense of control.

—∞—

Dependability is my greatest caregiving asset, and I'm proud of it.

—∞—

I'm not afraid to revise my task list when necessary.

Creativity is an important part of each caregiving day.

—⁂—

Instead of haste, a slow and steady caregiving approach
usually works best.

—⁂—

Modifying a home for caregiving may become a work in progress.

—⁂—

Conducting regular home assessments helps to keep my loved one safe.

—⁂—

As I go about my daily tasks, I try not to be hard on myself, and I cut
myself some slack.

—⁂—

To reduce stress, I avoid tight, demanding schedules.

All caregivers have hectic days, and when this happens
I consciously calm my mind.

—⚭—

Demanding as the daily routine may be, having a routine
is better than none.

—⚭—

Written reminders help me and my loved one, and I use them often.

—⚭—

Grocery lists, health care lists, and To Do lists help me manage
my caregiving.

—⚭—

To manage my time, I keep a neat house and prioritize tasks.

—⚭—

Experience can be a harsh teacher, yet I remember the
caregiving lessons.

Categorizing concerns (loved one's health, money, legal documents,
training, communication, personal health)
is the first problem-solving step.

—⁂—

Limiting discussion to one topic at a time improves
caregiver-receiver communication.

—⁂—

Linking the older generation with the younger is a permanent goal.

—⁂—

Writing a caregiving job description helps me clarify my
thinking and tasks.

—⁂—

Spoken and written words affirm my caregiving.

—⁂—

I apply my innate talents to caregiving.

It isn't enough to think about caregiving; I act on my best thoughts.

—⁓—

Laws change, and updating a will is a good thing to do.

—⁓—

I understand that men may approach caregiving differently than women.

—⁓—

Choices are part of each day, and I make them by answering the question, "What's best for my loved one?"

—⁓—

Long-term caregiving has taught me how to conserve my energy.

—⁓—

I inform paid caregivers of changes in routines and medical appointments.

Family dynamics factor into caregiving, and I take them into consideration.

—w—

Since I can't be all things to all family members, I don't even try.

—w—

Caregiving may well be the hardest job I've had in my life.

—w—

Caregiving and household schedules don't always mesh; so be it.

—w—

Caregiving tasks include updating the daily routine.

—w—

Every age and stage of life has its losses, and I am preparing for them.

A chronically ill or debilitated care receiver may become self-absorbed, and this requires extra patience.

—◊◊—

Education helps with caregiving, but it doesn't immunize me against the pain of watching my loved one struggle.

—◊◊—

Since health care professionals know how to navigate the insurance maze, I ask for their help.

—◊◊—

I continue to add to my repertoire of caregiving skills.

—◊◊—

Juggling my caregiving life and personal life is a daily task.

—◊◊—

The first step in going around caregiving barriers is to identify them.

Some caregiving tasks are improvisational. What fun!

—⧓—

Having fun is our shared caregiving goal.

CHAPTER 2

Safeguarding Health

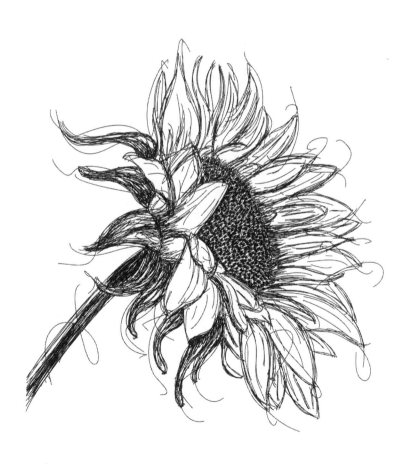

Learning about my loved one's disease/disability is an ongoing task,
and I benefit from it.

—◊—

Medical lingo is an important part of caregiving, and I learn
new words constantly.

—◊—

To keep my loved one safe, I stay informed on the side effects
of medications.

—◊—

I give my loved one medications as directed and renew prescriptions.

—◊—

Always, I credit my loved one for what he (she) can do.

—◊—

Caring for my loved one is like a prayer.

Fixing tasty, healthy meals for my loved one makes me feel good.

—⚏—

Monitoring snack foods and avoiding empty calories is
a savvy health decision.

—⚏—

Medical and dental checkups are an integral part of my caregiving
plans.

—⚏—

I keep notes and records pertaining to my loved one's health.

—⚏—

A daily checklist, printed each morning, helps me track
my loved one's medications.

—⚏—

Memory aids—a clock, calendar, photos, meaningful objects—help
my loved one retrieve mental data.

Working with a health care team requires effort, patience, and follow-up, three qualities I thankfully possess.

—ᴍ—

Visitors to the hospital's Intensive Care Unit, if they come often, slowly become a family, and that's comforting.

—ᴍ—

Our home has lots of health equipment, and while it is useful, the best equipment is a cheerful attitude.

—ᴍ—

The word "disability" means different things to different people.

—ᴍ—

Forgetfulness can be temporary, and I keep this in mind.

—ᴍ—

Setting some boundaries helps my loved one and me.

I'm glad adult day care is available for those who might benefit from it.

—ɯ—

There are two kinds of privacy, physical and mental, and I respect both.

—ɯ—

Thanks to mental spade work, my loved one identified his (her)
new life purpose.

—ɯ—

Each small success my loved one achieves is worthy of celebration.

—ɯ—

A loved one with memory problems can still say wise things.

—ɯ—

My loved one and I are growing old together, something we planned
from the first moment we met.

Staying fit for my age is my caregiver's goal.

———

To protect my loved one from infection, I wash my hands often and wear exam gloves.

———

If I don't ask, I won't know, so I ask health care professionals the questions that puzzle me.

———

The paid caregivers who come four hours a day keep me from compassion fatigue—physical and mental exhaustion.

———

Positive thinking reduces stress, improves health, makes me resistant to colds, improves coping skills, and, most surprising of all, prolongs my life.

———

If my loved one isn't feeling well, I cancel our plans and focus on his (her) health.

Good lighting is essential for safety, and I keep a supply of light bulbs on hand.

—⁂—

I make allowances for institutionalization—an overdependence on caregivers, intense focus on self, and treating family like staff.

—⁂—

I thought I knew my loved one well, yet caregiving has revealed new facets of personality and character.

—⁂—

Consulting a physician before ordering a wheelchair is a wise move.

—⁂—

Working with health care teams is a privilege and a responsibility.

—⁂—

Chronic illness has a ripple effect on the family, and I cope with these effects.

Catastrophic illness has two victims; care receiver and caregiver.

—◊—

I treat health care professionals the way I want to be treated, with courtesy, kindness, and respect.

—◊—

I respect my loved one's need for modesty.

—◊—

Signs of forgetfulness are things to record in writing.

—◊—

My loved one's medication history affects his (her) mind, and I stay current on this history.

—◊—

Thanks to advance planning, my loved one's room doesn't look like a hospital room; it looks like a bedroom.

National health organizations and their local chapters are reliable sources of information.

—❦—

Rehabilitation progress is measured in fractions of an inch, and each fraction, no matter how tiny, is significant.

—❦—

Excessive anesthesia can diminish a loved one's sense of taste, and I make allowances for this.

—❦—

Storing prescription medications and over-the-counter medications separately saves time.

—❦—

I check the dates of all medications and dispose of expired ones.

—❦—

We follow hospital procedures—no visitors when medications are being given or when a health care agency representative is present.

My loved one may have more than one illness, and that's why
I arrange for follow-up checkups.

—⚬⚬⚬—

Visitors are welcome unless they have a cold, are in the throes of a cold,
or are recovering from one.

—⚬⚬⚬—

For safety, I make sure the physician's order matches the order
on the medication bottle.

—⚬⚬⚬—

I accompany my loved one to rehabilitation sessions, not just to cheer
for him (her), but to witness the miracles that are taking place.

—⚬⚬⚬—

Years ago, the saltshaker was removed from our table,
and we are healthier for it.

—⚬⚬⚬—

Because I may need to contact a health care professional,
I keep all the business cards that I receive.

Number one on my caregiving plan: locate the nearest hospital, drive there, and note how long it takes.

—⚬—

The contact information for my loved one's primary care physician is handy.

—⚬—

As a patient advocate, I represent my loved one's wishes and accept the responsibilities that come with this role.

—⚬—

I love it when the seasons change and I can give my loved one different fruits and vegetables.

—⚬—

Serving meals at regular times helps my loved one and me maintain our energy and health.

—⚬—

As I learn more about my loved one's health issues, I am awed by his (her) ability to adapt.

My loved one's desire for independence is really courage at work.

CHAPTER 3

Making the Most of Every Day

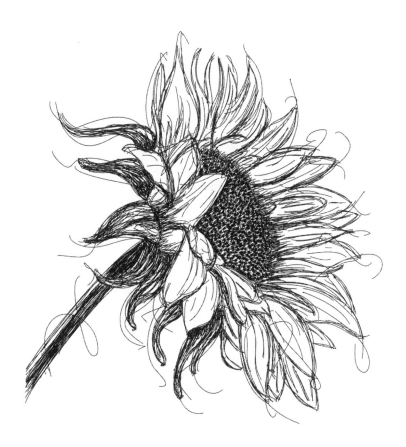

Mornings can get off to a rocky start, and to improve my mood,
I think of three people who have made my life better.

—⚏—

Reviewing plans in the morning helps the day go smoothly.

—⚏—

Special times—dinner with relatives, watching birds at the feeders,
reading in front of the fire—enrich my caregiving days.

—⚏—

I do my best each day and go to bed secure in this knowledge.

—⚏—

Caring for my loved one is my new life mission, and it is sacred.

—⚏—

It's okay to surprise myself every now and then.

Day-to-day caregiving can be stressful, so I build de-stressors
into my schedule.

—⟋⟍—

A brief break from caregiving renews my energy for days.

—⟋⟍—

Sometimes I leave for an hour or so and spend time with friends.

—⟋⟍—

Laughter is part of each caregiving day, and I'm not afraid
to laugh at myself.

—⟋⟍—

There is a sameness to caregiving days, yet I bring
original ideas to them.

—⟋⟍—

Spousal caregiving is different, so I identify problems quickly, discuss
them with my loved one, and take steps to solve these problems.

I posted a caregiver's prayer on the refrigerator and read it often.

———

Setbacks are a chance to review, rest, and evaluate caregiving.

———

I know kindness and caregiving are more important than being right.

———

From the first moment of the day to the last, I respect my loved one's experience and dignity.

———

Sometimes I have to go backward in order to move forward.

———

There are no perfect caregivers or perfect caregiving days, and that's that!

I can't control life events, but I can control my responses to them.

—⁓—

I admit it: some days I think I'm losing my mind, though I'm not.

—⁓—

Unexpected gifts bring unexpected joy.

—⁓—

When things get tough, I say, "I love you."

—⁓—

As time passes, I become more aware of the types of stress I experience.

—⁓—

"You should" is often a negative statement, and when I hear it
I tend to tune out.

I'm grateful for the miracle of life and am aware of living the miracle.

A smile from my loved one transforms the day.

In early morning, when the moon is still shining and it is barely light,
I center my thoughts and greet the dawn.

Keeping a journal is a creative way to problem-solve.

Dependence can be a challenging situation, and my loved one's
dependence honors me.

Caregiving may be the last time to discuss family issues,
and I make the most of this time.

Just like my loved one, I have needs, am aware of them,
and work on them.

—⚹—

Overthinking an issue doesn't guarantee a savvy decision.

—⚹—

Assessing my skills honestly helps me see what I need and get support.

—⚹—

Annoyance is an annoying feeling, and I work hard to get rid of it.

—⚹—

As I go about my day, I'm aware of my talents and limitations.

—⚹—

When I feel sorry for myself, I think of caregivers who are
coping with greater challenges than mine.

Ambiguity can be confusing and delay caregiving progress.

—∞—

Attentiveness requires energy and concentration;
it is a gift for my loved one.

—∞—

Some friends stay in touch, while others drift away,
and I understand this.

—∞—

Some things that happen are out of my control,
and acknowledgement is the only "solution."

—∞—

Endurance counts when it comes to caregiving.

—∞—

Caregiving has altered my housekeeping, and things like
not making the bed don't upset me anymore.

No matter what happens in a day, I still say "yes" to life.

—⚏—

"Work keeps me sane," a friend said, and I get it.

—⚏—

A contingency plan is a necessary part of caregiving,
and I keep ours current.

—⚏—

When things go wrong, I don't expect to be rescued; I rescue myself.

—⚏—

I don't do things the way my loved one would do them, but they get
done, and that's what really matters.

—⚏—

Endings are often beginnings, and I remind myself of this often.

When my loved one is having a bad day, I need to have a good day.

—◊—

I avoid chronic complainers and seek chronic boosters.

—◊—

Becoming a caregiver has led to new and beneficial friendships.

—◊—

Time management skills come from experience, practice, and the willingness to try new things; and I'm willing to try.

—◊—

Until I wrote our schedule on paper, I didn't understand its scope. No wonder I get tired.

—◊—

Paid caregivers are helpful, but I'm the person responsible for making the final decisions.

Keeping a caregiving happiness jar, filled with notes about happy moments of the day, documents my life and brings me joy.

—〰—

Laughter helps me let go of problems for a little while.

—〰—

Tomorrow gives me the chance to begin anew.

—〰—

Caregiving is my new job, in addition to all the others I have, and I like them all.

—〰—

I'm aware of my secondary losses, things like less time with friends, and try to accommodate them.

—〰—

Worries can come in clusters, but I focus on one worry at a time.

When I'm home, I often sing to myself because I'm happy.
Yes, I give myself "high fives" for the tasks I've done well.

—∿—

At bedtime, I put negatives aside and review the positives of my
caregiving day.

—∿—

Reading, a love I developed early in childhood, is a respite for
body and mind.

—∿—

Reading poetry quiets my mind and leads to peace of mind.

—∿—

I seek silence, a wellspring of strength, caregiving ideas,
and solutions to problems.

—∿—

Quiet caregiving days are some of the best.

CHAPTER 4

Loving My Loved One

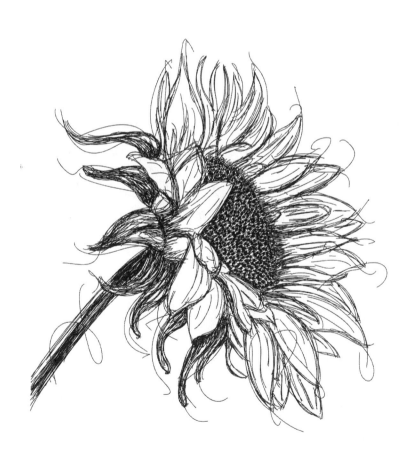

Caregiving is a journey, and love is my guide.

———

My loved one and I are a caregiving team—small but mighty.

———

I constantly learn from my loved one, and that is a blessing.

———

Reversing roles is part of caregiving, and some days my loved one encourages me more than I encourage him (her).

———

Pictures are hung lower than usual so my loved one can see them from his (her) wheelchair.

———

My loved one's sweet nature makes caregiving easier.

Seeing my loved one struggle is painful, and then I realize,
yet again, it is a sign of courage.

—◆—

There is no better time to speak of love than now.

—◆—

Caring for my loved one gives me chances to make new memories.

—◆—

When patience wanes, I mentally reverse roles with my loved one
and ask, "How would I feel in this situation?"

—◆—

When I have to say no, I say it gently.

—◆—

I compliment my loved one every chance I get.

Short compliments are easier for my loved one to remember.

———

Small blessings, such as my loved one saying, "Thanks so much," make caregiving special.

———

The smell of baking cookies makes our house feel like home, and my loved one can hardly wait to taste a cookie.

———

Family history is important, so I encourage my loved one to put his (her) experiences in writing.

———

Depression can be anger with nowhere to go, and I monitor my loved one for symptoms of depression.

———

My loved one's smile is always a gift.

Even if I've heard the story many times, I smile and listen to my loved one's story again.

—⁓—

Being home with my loved one, working quietly while he (she) reads, makes me happy.

—⁓—

Silence is a form of communication, and it's one I use.

—⁓—

Hard as it is, I resist the urge to be overprotective and, instead, foster my loved one's independence.

—⁓—

It's fun to surprise my loved one with a new magazine or book, especially when he (she) is so grateful.

—⁓—

Love is my caregiving song, and it plays all the time.

"I will not fail you" is a pledge to my loved one and a promise
to myself.

—◊—

When my patience wanes, I spell "l-o-v-e" in my mind
to restore patience.

—◊—

My loved one is my champion, and I am his (hers).

—◊—

I melt inside when my loved one declares, "Good for you!"

—◊—

Caring for a disabled loved one requires extra planning
because tasks take twice as much time to complete.

—◊—

I will always be part of my loved one's cheering section.

Hearing loss complicates caregiving, and I work around it, speaking slowly, repeating sentences, and facing my loved one when I speak.

—ᴡ—

Before I make a major purchase, I consult my loved one.

—ᴡ—

Because every moment is precious, we strive to do things together, even if it requires extra effort.

—ᴡ—

My loved one is my hero (heroine) and always will be.

—ᴡ—

Keeping my loved one safe is a continuous goal.

—ᴡ—

Things can happen for no reason, and asking myself, "Why did this happen?" can be a waste of time.

Being my loved one's advocate requires truthfulness,
and I'm always truthful.

—⚬—

I proceed according to my loved one's needs, not based
on what others think.

—⚬—

Saturday evenings have become date nights, times to
enjoy some wine and reflect on our lives.

—⚬—

Caregiving has made our love stronger than it has ever been.

—⚬—

Each day, my loved one and I are making history.

—⚬—

Caring for my loved one has given me new challenges
and unexpected happiness.

There are times when no words are needed and love speaks for me.

—⚭—

Due to my loved one's disability, we moved to a one-level home, and,
upsetting as this was, we've landed safely.

—⚭—

Furnished with things from the past, our new place looks like us
and feels like home.

—⚭—

Despite his (her) physical challenges, my loved one has goals
and works toward them.

—⚭—

When my loved one is frustrated, I touch his (her) hand and say,
"We're lucky to be here together."

—⚭—

The love that shines from my loved one's eyes renews
my sense of purpose.

Laughter is just one of the ties that bind us together.

—⚏—

Caregiving works because of love.

—⚏—

The values my loved one and I share are still our values,
and we live by them.

—⚏—

The loneliness of caregiving is softened by the love we have
for one another.

—⚏—

I benefit daily from my loved one's wisdom.

—⚏—

My loved one and I know each other so well we think the same things
and speak the same sentences.

Knowing I am deeply loved is a gift I will cherish forever.

—◊◊◊—

Caregiving has given the word "love" new meaning.

—◊◊◊—

We talk about our experiences, each with a different view;
my loved one, the scientist who remembers highway routes, and me,
the creative person who remembers shapes and colors.

—◊◊◊—

Only now, with the clarity of hindsight, do we realize that
both of us have had extraordinary lives.

CHAPTER 5

Taking Care of Me

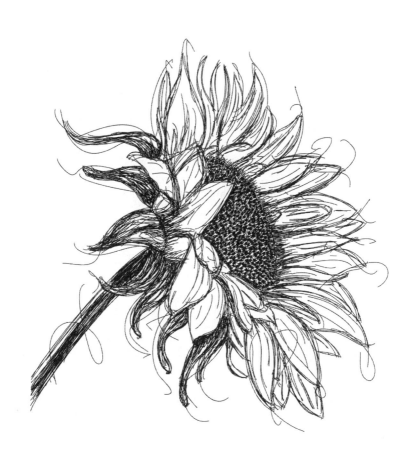

For my health and wellbeing, I choose to spend time with upbeat, positive people.

—⚭—

Noise contributes to stress, and that's why I have a quiet reading place.

—⚭—

Being hard on myself accomplishes nothing; practicing self-compassion gives me a burst of energy.

—⚭—

As I care for my loved one, I am aware of my own physical limitations and accommodate them.

—⚭—

Walking helps me stay physically fit, and I walk around every grocery store aisle three times on inclement days.

—⚭—

It's amazing how a fifteen-minute walk helps me de-stress.

Self-care is part of caregiving, and I take good care of myself.

—⁓—

"I will not neglect my health" is a promise I make to myself each day.

—⁓—

Joining a caregiving support group is one of the best decisions
I ever made.

—⁓—

Friends offer suggestions, but I'm the one in the caregiving trenches,
making my way each day.

—⁓—

We stay connected to others by donating to community organizations.

—⁓—

I'm responsible for my happiness, nobody else—not family, not friends,
not other caregivers.

Caring for a disabled person can be sad, so I stay alert to the symptoms of anticipatory grief.

—⁊⁊—

"Me time," a few quiet minutes to myself, is a part of each caregiving day.

—⁊⁊—

Doing something for myself each day helps me retain my sense of self.

—⁊⁊—

An hour nap refreshes me for the rest of the day.

—⁊⁊—

Every so often, I have a lazy day to renew my energy and caregiving perspective.

—⁊⁊—

I watch for symptoms of compassion fatigue—poor sleep, forgetfulness, grouchiness, lethargy, emotional numbness—because I don't want this for myself.

Self-compassion is an antidote to compassion fatigue.

—∿—

When I feel overwhelmed, I ask for help.

—∿—

Asking for help isn't a sign of weakness; it is a reality check.

—∿—

I continue to do things that make me happy.

—∿—

Keeping social contacts is difficult, but I continue to work at it.

—∿—

Having a bedtime ritual helps me prepare for sleep and sleep well.

One friend can get me though a challenging day.

———

Support group meetings aren't complaint sessions;
they are opportunities to share personal stories and
learn from other caregivers.

———

I continue to work on accepting the things I cannot change.

———

Limiting television news programs is a form of self-protection.

———

Tiredness creeps up on me, and when this happens I tell myself,
"I can do this."

———

Caring for my spiritual self helps me be a better caregiver.

I became a caregiver willingly and lovingly, but it doesn't define me
as a person.

—⟋⟍—

Breaking out of the isolation bubble takes courage,
and I'm doing it little by little.

—⟋⟍—

Since the majority of caregivers are women, I listen attentively
when I chat with a male caregiver.

—⟋⟍—

New experiences are energizing, and I seek them out.

—⟋⟍—

Fear can cause worry, but, more importantly, it can lead to action.

—⟋⟍—

Some aspects of caregiving are sad, and I work to contain my sadness.

Delaying a decision can be a form of denial, and I need to
be aware of this.

—〰—

I take care of my health so I can care for my loved one.

—〰—

The energy of a hearty laugh can't be measured, but it can be felt.

—〰—

Offers of help are touching, but I am selective about accepting them.

—〰—

Caregiving makes me aware of my limitations,
something I need to know.

—〰—

To manage stress, some keep a God box—a box to store worries
written on paper—and turn these worries over to God.

Busy as my life is, I continue to learn and challenge my intelligence.

—⁂—

Written words, whether they are affirmations, journal entries, or emails, reveal surprising things about caregiving.

—⁂—

Silence is a necessary part of caregiving life; it helps me clarify ideas and plan for the future.

—⁂—

Because regrets are non-productive, I choose to focus on caregiving successes.

—⁂—

Without self-care and personal growth, caregiving becomes merely existing.

—⁂—

"Who am I now?" is a question many caregivers ask, including me, and it's a logical question.

A family caregiver is always prepared for a change of plans;
at least, that's what I tell myself.

—⟋⟍—

I refuse to let fatigue dilute my caregiving resolve.

—⟋⟍—

Obstacles can be a sign of progress, not regression,
and that is comforting.

—⟋⟍—

Restful sleep is food for the body and the soul.

—⟋⟍—

I'm a link in the caregiving chain, and connecting with other caregivers
makes my link stronger.

—⟋⟍—

As the supply of paid caregivers decreases, the demand for them
increases, and this makes me ask, "Who will care for me?"

"No" is often a self-care word, one I use to defend myself and my time.

—⁂—

A funny Internet video can keep me laughing all day.

—⁂—

When I am upset, I discuss my feelings with my loved one
and always feel better.

—⁂—

It's hard, some days, to tell who is taking greater care;
my loved one or me.

—⁂—

Love is a balm that soothes the aches and pains of life.

—⁂—

I turn down friends' offers to grocery shop for me because shopping
is my "outing" and I need the break.

Because I love to bake, I make time for it, and I always enjoy
the experience.

—⚊—

Caregiving involves fairness for the care receiver and fairness
for the caregiver.

—⚊—

Five minutes of meditation helps me slow racing thoughts
and calm my soul.

—⚊—

After a frigid winter, I watch for seasonal changes and the first robin,
a harbinger of spring.

—⚊—

I accept the responsibilities of caregiving and accept additional
responsibilities because I care.

—⚊—

I'm an organized person, and when I feel like it I schedule "nothing
days"— times when I do as little as possible and recharge my batteries.

Whether I'm peppy or tired, happy or sad, ready or not,
my mind is always working.

—⚏—

When I have a creative idea, I follow the leads and see where they go.

—⚏—

Common sense often answers my caregiving questions,
and I trust mine.

—⚏—

In the long run, helping other caregivers helps me.

CHAPTER 6

Words of Emotional Support

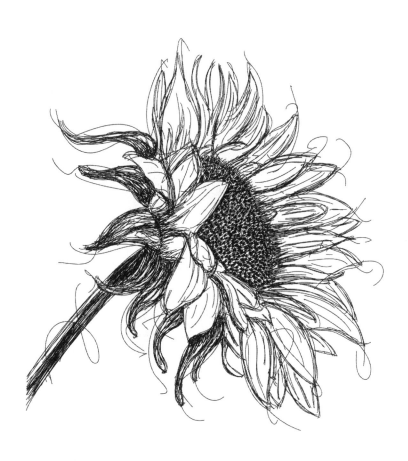

When I start to feel down, I go back in time and revive
happy memories.

—⟐—

Becoming a caregiver is a way of giving back for all the love, care,
and encouragement I've received.

—⟐—

Sharing experiences with other family caregivers makes me feel
less alone.

—⟐—

When I feel isolated, I make an effort to connect with others.

—⟐—

Some days it is best to keep negative thoughts to myself;
tomorrow will be better.

—⟐—

Compliments on my cooking always make me feel good.

Self-compassion—a combination of kindness, respect for others, and mindful living—is something I work on constantly.

—⁓—

I deal with negative feelings by identifying their sources, learning more, and taking proactive steps.

—⁓—

Positive thinking, even if I have to work hard at it, helps my loved one and me.

—⁓—

When problems seem overwhelming, I give myself an attitude adjustment.

—⁓—

People say I'm their hero; I'm not a hero, I'm a wife, mother, and grandmother who takes care of those I love.

—⁓—

Dwelling on the past is a waste of time, so I focus my eyes on the present.

Each of us—caregiver and receiver—is entitled to our feelings.

—⚏—

Sometimes I cry because I care so much.

—⚏—

At one time or another, a caregiver gets angry,
and I divert the energy of anger to something good.

—⚏—

Giving to others makes me feel good from the top of my head to the
soles of my feet.

—⚏—

Mindful living, an acute awareness of my body and what is happening
at the moment, is a challenge worthy of effort.

—⚏—

Keeping a happiness jar, filled with dated messages about happy
experiences, helps me see life positively and appreciate the life I have.

I face my feelings and take the time to name them.

—∾—

In the quiet times of the day, I hear my thoughts and soul in action.

—∾—

Though I have a new job, I'm still me, and I take steps
to retain my identity.

—∾—

If I am patient, work hard, and persist,
happiness can grow from sadness.

—∾—

Self-confidence is a gift to myself, and I give it often.

—∾—

Letting go is a gradual process, one I am working on,
and it includes letting go of unfulfilled dreams.

Family members don't have to agree on everything in order
to provide support.

———

Smiling leads to positive thoughts, and I have a lot to smile about.

———

Laughter lifts my spirits and, as time passes,
helps me develop resilience.

———

When I disagree with someone, I speak in a moderate voice
and pitch to ensure my message is received.

———

Confronting fear is better than pushing scary thoughts
to the back of my mind.

———

Though I don't know how long my caregiving journey will be
or where it will lead, I still enjoy the journey.

Occasionally, I am resentful and realize this feeling is normal.

—❧—

Caregiving has its own rhythm, and I hear the beat.

—❧—

Reading caregiving books helps me and makes me aware
of my unique situation.

—❧—

I have a circle of support, and it is getting larger.

—❧—

Silly mistakes can generate self-anger, an uncomfortable feeling
that I address.

—❧—

Essential supplies—a gentle spirit and heart—are always with me.

Emotional checkups—identifying feelings and naming them—
help me stay on course.

—◊—

Because I've received support, I support other caregivers personally,
online, or via email.

—◊—

Laughter is common at our house, and I reap its benefits.

—◊—

As the months pass, my caregiving days become more precious.

—◊—

Surely I'm not the only caregiver who talks to herself (himself);
besides, I'm an interesting person.

—◊—

After months of experience and study, some caregiving duties
still surprise me.

Inner peace begins with me and my yearning for it.

—ɷ—

An upsetting experience doesn't destroy my day;
I simply choose happiness again.

—ɷ—

I view caregiving as an adventure, and I'm part of it.

—ɷ—

My caregiving is unique, and although I know other caregivers,
I don't compare myself to them.

—ɷ—

Sometimes decision-making comes down to trusting my instincts,
and I have good ones.

—ɷ—

Work can be a source of emotional support: but it can also
be avoidance, something I don't need.

Music stays in my mind for weeks, and when it plays in my mind,
my spirits soar.

———

British poet Sir Edward Dyer wrote about his mind being his kingdom.
My mind is often my kingdom, and I am surprised at what I see.

———

I finally learned how to accept compliments,
and I'm glad I learned this.

———

Because I'm a visual person, I keep lists of words that lift my spirits:
tender, gentle, kind, caring, funny, and others.

———

Color influences mood, so I try to wear happy colors.

———

Amazing how a haircut can make me feel good all day.

When a friend said, "You look happy," I realized how happy I am.

—ɯ—

Smiling lifts my mood and the mood of those I meet.

—ɯ—

Watching flowers bud and bloom always makes me happy.

CHAPTER 7

Celebrating the Positives

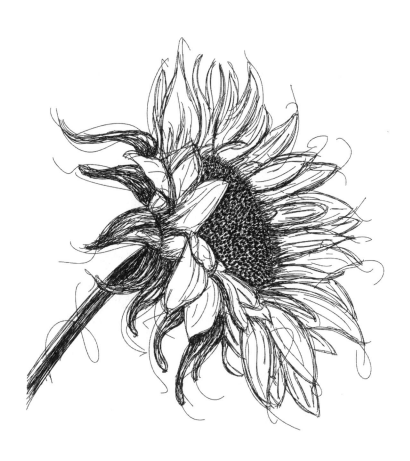

Hope comes in baby steps, yet they lead me forward.

———

Optimism is as contagious as the common cold, thank goodness.

———

When another caregiver starts to complain,
I change the topic and talk about positive things.

———

I keep a caregiving journal for myself, family members,
and generations to come.

———

I'm aware of the preciousness of these days, and I savor them.

———

New drugs and surgical procedures are invented constantly,
and this gives me hope.

My supportive family and extended family are ongoing sources of hope.

———

Positive self-talk boosts my spirits.

———

Family members are adjusting to the caregiving situation, and so am I.

———

Religious and spiritual beliefs are sources of support,
and I'm grateful for them.

———

Writing can be done anywhere, and I'm blessed to be able
to work at home.

———

The flame of hope may be small, but it still exists,
and I do all I can to keep the candle burning.

Becoming a caregiver has made me a more sensitive person.

———

Online communities provide information and support.

———

Caregiving gives me the chance to meet new people,
make new friends, and learn new things.

———

Older adults still set goals, and I'm one of these adults.

———

Good news: depression in older adults isn't a "given."

———

It's simple: If I'm courteous to others, I am usually treated
courteously.

Attending support group meetings helps me put life in perspective and realize that others face far greater challenges than I do.

—⧞—

Humor can diffuse a difficult situation and open the way to negotiation.

—⧞—

The fear of hoping too much doesn't stop me from hoping.

—⧞—

Though I don't know what the future holds, I do know I'll make the most of my days.

—⧞—

Happiness is a choice, and I choose it for myself every day.

—⧞—

Patience may be courage in disguise.

Time has taught me an important lesson—creating a new normal
can be exciting.

—⚬⚬—

Most of my self-talk is positive because I make it so.

—⚬⚬—

Body language is a form of communication,
and I've learned to read it well.

—⚬⚬—

Love is a beacon of hope and lights my way.

—⚬⚬—

Blooming flowers in our home are sources of color and conversation.

—⚬⚬—

Today there are far more resources for family caregivers than
there were ten years ago. Hooray!

I always do my best, for these days will never come again.

—ᗰ—

Improving my listening skills has helped me with other life experiences.

—ᗰ—

Caregiving may determine the success of my life,
and I'm okay with that.

—ᗰ—

In one of his poems, Robert Frost says some things need to
"take their course," and hope is one of these things.

—ᗰ—

At every caregiving support meeting I get ideas from other caregivers
that may work for me.

—ᗰ—

Remembering my mission—to care for, protect, and love my loved one
more each day—helps with decision-making.

Confidence comes from experience, and experience comes
from loving care.

—⚒—

My approach is to do what I can when I can, and it works well.

—⚒—

The physical demands of caregiving—bending, lifting, reaching,
stretching—are helping to keep me fit.

—⚒—

All caregivers have discouraging days, and when this happens,
I think about the rewards of caregiving.

—⚒—

Many caregivers quit their jobs to care for a loved one,
and I'm glad I can work at home.

—⚒—

Caregiving is love in action, and I do this out of love.

As the caregiving years pass, my love continues to grow.

—⟋⟍—

I laugh at my own jokes, and that's funny by itself.

—⟋⟍—

My loved one would care for me if the situation were reversed,
and I know this.

—⟋⟍—

Understanding friends are pillars of support,
and their understanding continues.

—⟋⟍—

Although love can't be measured, it lasts forever.

—⟋⟍—

Each caregiving day is a day of discovery.

The art of caregiving is honed by experience,
and I gain experience daily.

—ɯ—

Taking the time to know myself makes me a better caregiver.

—ɯ—

Hobbies help me relax and this forges resilience.

—ɯ—

My loved one can live a high-quality life even though he (she) is in
a wheelchair.

—ɯ—

My loved one's therapists are so dedicated, giving, and determined
that it brings tears to my eyes.

—ɯ—

Caregiving is challenging, and though I'm a grandmother,
I still love a good challenge.

I still have more to give and am exploring ways to do it.

—⚋—

Being a caregiver affirms my life; I am loved and needed.

—⚋—

Family members continue to support, comfort, and help me.

—⚋—

Because we create it together, caregiving is a gift for my loved one and myself.

—⚋—

At night, when I go to sleep, I smile because I've spent another precious day with my loved one.

—⚋—

Words can stay in the mind for years, so I choose my words carefully and lovingly.

Reading an affirmation a day keeps the blues at bay.

———

I can write my own affirmations. Woo-hoo!

CHAPTER 8

Affirming Myself with Words

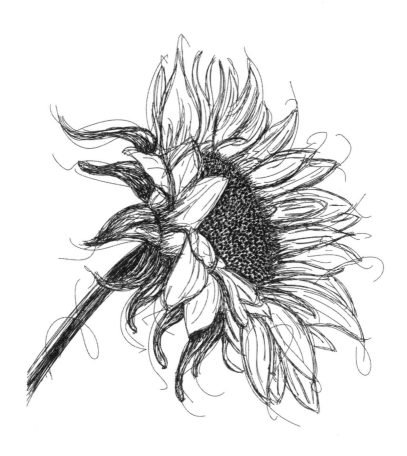

Benefits of Affirmation Writing

Doctors, health care providers, and counselors recommend affirmation writing because it works. Putting your thoughts in writing validates your ideas, makes them real, and can change your outlook in seconds. Here are some of the other benefits:

You think positively. As you write an affirmation, negative thoughts may come to mind. Instead of focusing on negatives, you focus on positives. For example, rather than writing "Caregiving is exhausting," you may write "Caregiving gives me opportunities to know my loved one better."

This kind of writing is proactive. You are expressing your innermost thoughts and taking care of yourself. As your list of affirmations grows, you become more aware of the positives in your life. Over time, affirmation writing becomes an empowering experience.

Making word choices clears mental clutter. You have to make word choices when you write affirmations, and this process helps you sort your thoughts. Negative words are discarded and replaced by positive ones, such as **kindness**, **caring**, and **love**.

Affirmation writing is quick. A journal requires regular entries and a diary requires daily entries—both lots of work. In contrast, affirmation writing takes only a few minutes. Writing affirmations regularly may become a form of self-help.

You can write affirmations anywhere. An affirmation may come to mind when you're driving, shopping for groceries, doing the dishes, or watching television. The minute you think of it, write the affirmation on a pad, scratch paper, an old envelope, a cash register receipt—anything that's handy. Later in the day, you may wish to enter this affirmation into your computer file.

Affirmations may become goals. Some of your affirmations may be expressions of what you hope will happen. Over time, with work and persistence, you make these affirmations come true. When you write affirmations, you discover surprising things about yourself and see caregiving more clearly. These results are worth your time and effort.

Affirmation Writing Tips

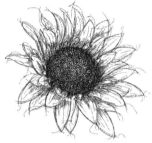

- Find a comfortable place to sit, and eliminate all background noise, if possible.

- Slow your thoughts and clear the clutter from your mind. Visualizing a blank television screen may help you to do this.

- Think of something positive in your life. It can be a small thing, such as making delicious coffee.

- Create an affirmation about your positive thought. If you can't write a sentence, write one word, such as *love* or *grateful*.

- Use the present tense. Affirm the caregiving life you are living now. After you have done this, move on to writing affirmations about the life you hope to have.

- Check your affirmation for tone and word choices. Tweak it a little if you must, but resist the urge to overwork your affirmation.

- Write one-sentence affirmations. They are easier to remember and easier to jot down on a small piece of paper to stick in your pocket.

- Keep writing affirmations, and read them aloud from time to time.

- Watch for forward steps in your life journey. Dating your affirmations will help you track them.

- Apply your affirmations to everyday life.

Practice Pages

Start writing some affirmations here. You may expand on affirmations in this book or go in new directions. Use the next page and continue to write affirmations when they come to mind.

_____

_____

_____

_____

_____

_____

_____

_____

_____

_____

_____

_____

Another page for your affirmations.

_____

_____

_____

_____

_____

_____

_____

_____

_____

_____

_____

_____

_____

_____

_____

_____

About the Author

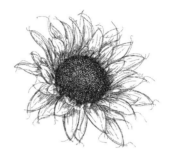

Harriet Hodgson has been a freelance writer for more than thirty-six years and is the author of thirty-five books and thousands of print and Internet articles. She is a member of the Association of Health Care Journalists, Association for Death Education and Counseling, and Minnesota Coalition for Death Education and Support. In addition, she is a contributing writer for The Caregiver Space website, Open to Hope Foundation website, and The Grief Toolbox website.

She has appeared on more than 180 radio talk shows, blog talk radio, and dozens of television stations, including CNN. A popular speaker, Hodgson has given presentations at public health, Alzheimer's, and bereavement conferences. Currently, she is giving talks to community groups about caregiving, creating a happy life, and a writing life. Her work is cited in *Who's Who of American Women, World Who's Who of Women, Contemporary Authors*, and other author directories.

Hodgson lives in Rochester, Minnesota, with her husband, John. Please visit **www.harriethodgson.com** for more information about this busy author, wife, and grandmother.

Also by Harriet Hodgson

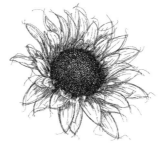

The Family Caregiver's Guide,
available from www.writelife.com, Amazon, and bookstores.

Happy Again! Your New and Meaningful Life After Loss,
available from www.writelife.com, Amazon, and bookstores.

*Alzheimer's: Finding the Words, A Communication Guide for
Those Who Care*,
available from John Wiley & Sons and Amazon.

Smiling Through Your Tears: Anticipating Grief,
with co-author Lois Krahn, MD, available from Amazon.

The Spiritual Woman: Quotes to Refresh and Sustain Your Soul,
available from Centering Corporation.

*101 Affirmations to Ease Your Grief Journey: Words of Comfort,
Words of Hope*, available from Amazon.

Seed Time: Growing from Life's Disappointments, Losses, and Sorrows,
available from Amazon.

Walking Woman: Step-by-Step to a Healthier Heart,
available from Amazon.